HEALTHY WEIGHT LOSS
IN THE
NEW YEAR

Lose Those Holiday Pounds

Without Dieting or Starving Yourself!

Ron Kness

Published by:

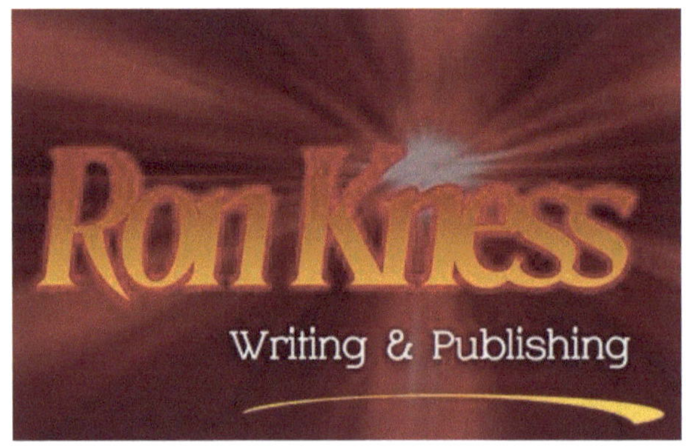

https://ronknesswriting.com

Ron Kness

Gold Canyon, AZ

United States of America

ISBN: 9781791781842

CONTENTS

INTRODUCTION

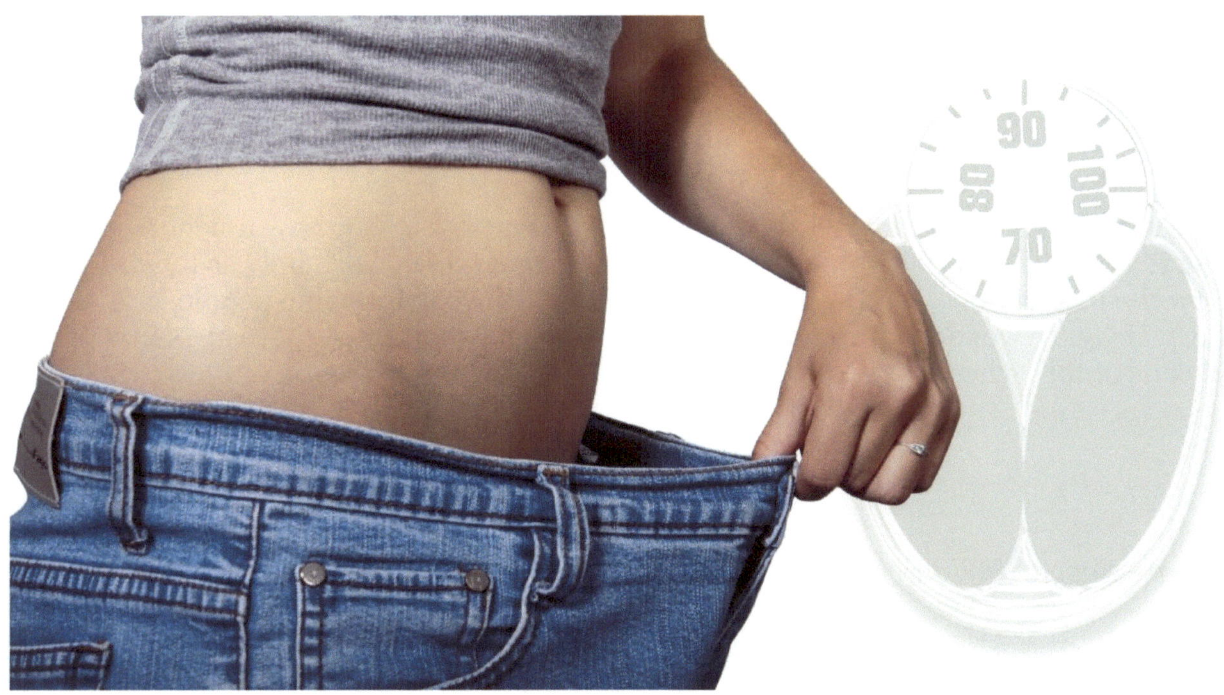

Losing weight is probably the most popular goal or New Years' resolution people make between December and January. While weight loss makes sense not just from an aesthetic perspective, but a health one as well, most diets and New Years' Resolutions based around dieting will fail.

This book will help you with losing weight in the New Year but it does take a different approach than most other weight loss techniques. It will talk about throwing conventional diets out the window and finding a healthier way to lose weight and keep it off … for good.

WHY DIETS DON'T WORK

This can be a hard pill to swallow, and possibly one of the hardest parts of accepting this type of weight loss "method". While diets do work for many people in the short-term, the chance of them allowing for long-term weight loss, where you keep it off, is slim to none.

There are many reasons for this, from having restrictions that lead to binge eating, to how unrealistic it is to have so many rules about what you can and can't eat. The fact is, if you want to lose weight in the healthiest way possible, you might want to reconsider being on a structured diet.

A structured diet is one that tells you what to eat, what not to eat, how much to eat, and when to eat. It is easy to say all diets don't work, or that diets work only as long as you follow the instructions, but the simple fact is that they work for some people, and not others. If you're wondering about the best approach to weight loss, here are some pros and cons of following a more structured diet.

Pros:

They are Easy to Follow

One of the reasons people like to do structured diets like Paleo, Keto, low-calorie, and others is because it tells you exactly what you need to do. This can make it a lot easier to follow in the beginning, especially when you feel like you want to start losing weight right away.

You Know All the Rules without Second Guessing Yourself

Similar to this is the fact that you don't have to spend a lot of time second guessing yourself. This is probably the number one reason people go for "diets" as opposed to just switching to making healthier food choices. You know exactly what to eat, what not to eat, how much to eat, and sometimes even when you should be eating.

It is Effective in the Short-Term

Structured diets are almost always effective, as long as you stick to the diet properly. If you want to start seeing those pounds come off now, this can be a good option for you. Just don't plan to stay ion it for a long time.

Cons:

There are Bigger Restrictions

Naturally, the main disadvantage of a structured diet is that it is restrictive. You are usually given a list of foods you can eat, but also a list of foods you can't. This creates a label for certain foods, where suddenly they become bad for you, and that can have some long-term repercussions.

It Might Not Last Long-Term

While you will probably see results pretty quickly with these diets, the results might not last. Many people find that once they go back to their old way of eating, all the pounds come back on, sometimes more and they deal with binge cycles, and yo-yo dieting. This is why making a permanent lifestyle change is best if you want lasting results.

It Makes it Hard to Build a Healthy Relationship with Food

You also damage your relationship with food when you label certain foods "bad". Suddenly, everything you eat becomes a test, where you figure out if you can eat it or not, have guilt or shame when you give in to cravings, and might end up gaining instead of losing.

The choice is always going to be individual, as many people do find diets help them lose the weight and keep it off.

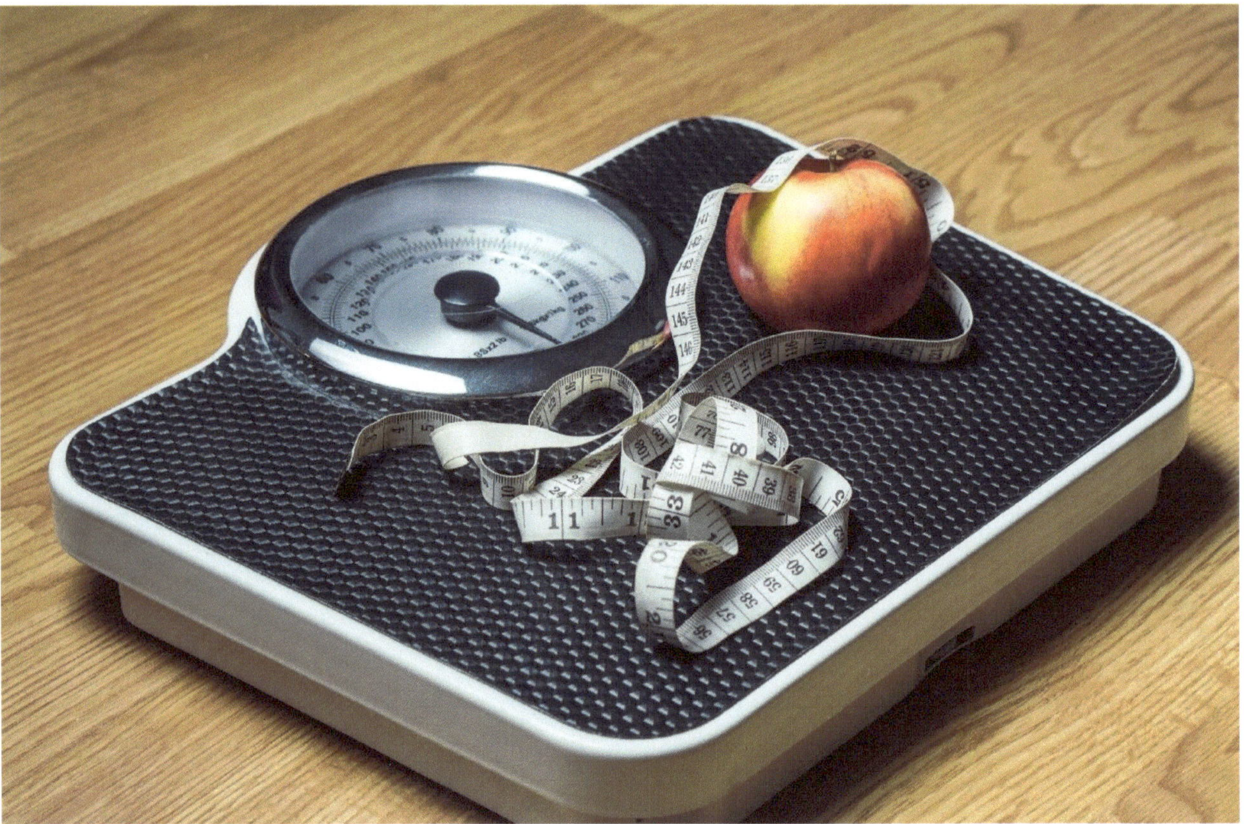

First of all, you are dealing with the diet mentality, which can be really harmful for not just your mental health, but your physical health as well. By being on a diet with rules about what you are eating, you are classifying certain foods or nutrients as "good" and "bad". Just by assigning this bad word to certain foods, you are creating a larger craving. Suddenly, you want nothing more than all these bad foods, even though before the diet, you would eat them only sparingly.

This is the diet mentality you want to break by giving up on these types of restrictive diets, and instead just focusing on fueling your body and staying nourished with the healthiest foods you can get your hands on.

Resulting Binge

Another thing that often happens when people go on diets is that they go through cyclical binges. You start off great, and almost get a type of high by sticking to your diet plan. You are sure this is going to be the one that helps you lose weight and keep it off for good.

But ultimately, you end up failing. There will come a day when you have a craving for the food you are told not to eat, and then you remind yourself you can't have it, which increases the craving. Eventually, you give in and have a full-out binge session.

Then you go back on the diet, possibly even more of a restrictive one to erase the damage you just did, and the cycle repeats itself.

Stopping the Cycle

The only way to stop this unhealthy cycle, get back on track, and lose weight for good is to ditch the diet mentality. Start focusing more on foods that are healthy and will nourish your body, and suddenly your entire mindset about food and weight will change dramatically.

And the best part? You will lose weight in a healthy, natural and lasting way, that doesn't feel difficult at all.

EAT HEALTHY WITHOUT STARVING

For a lot of people, the scariest thing about changing their eating habits is often the fear that they will have to endure days of feeling hungry and unsatisfied after meager meals. If this is one of the things that is keeping you from trying to eat healthy, then you'll be delighted to know that you'll have plenty of opportunity to feel completely full and satisfied when you eat the rights foods. The next few paragraphs will share a few ideas on how you can eat healthy without starving.

Soups Can Be Substantial

You might not think of soup as a big go to when you think of getting full, but that might be because you haven't seen many of the robust, hearty soups that are available to enjoy. If you look online you can find an array of recipes that incorporate rich, blended vegetable pastes, savory seasonings, literal medleys of vegetables, and many ideas that can include your favorite meats. Soups like these will not only fill you up but will probably make you feel like skipping the breads and other foods completely.

Apples, Oranges, and Bananas

It's easy to forget that nature has provided some efficient delivery systems for the essential nutrients that humans need to survive. Apples, oranges, and bananas can be placed in a carrier of some kind very easily and will keep well in most conditions. Bananas and apples are dense in flesh and contain large amounts of pectin which is great for your skin, and digestive system. They provide a decent amount of fiber as well, with will further aid with the cleanliness and efficiency of your digestion.

Broccoli and Other Greens

Thick cruciferous vegetables like broccoli are definitely your friend when it comes to those dinner-time meals. They contain a large amount of protein, fiber, potassium, a ton of antioxidants that come together to also aid in collagen production. Broccoli can be cooked and flavored in a variety of ways that make it a relatively versatile vegetable. You can even boil it for around 20 minutes until it becomes soft enough to whip into a thick soup.

Beans Are Filling

As the most underestimated of foods, beans are extremely tasty with basic seasoning, and they can be very filling. Well-made beans can be eaten with crackers or seed chips for a great snack, and with some added vegetables, they can become an entire meal. If you want to take it to the next level, then you can easily add a grain like rice to your beans and create an inexpensive yet healthy mixture that will keep well for at least 5 - 7 days. When rice and beans are eaten together they are a complete essential amino acid.

HOW THE ORDER OF WHAT YOU EAT MATTERS

Did you know the order of what you eat during each meal can actually make a difference? It changes everything, from how full you get and how quickly you get full, to how satiated you feel after your meal. This is great for anyone who tends to overeat, eat mindlessly, or almost always go for seconds or extra snacks after you have finished a meal.

Believe it or not, the order of what you eat on your plate does make a big difference. Here are some things to know about what order to eat what if you are trying to develop healthy eating habits, stop overeating, and start losing weight.

To Fill Up, Eat Protein First

If you find your appetite and overeating to be your biggest struggles when it comes to losing weight, you need to figure out how to feel fuller with each healthy meal you consume. To start with, eat your protein first! Protein is going to help keep you full and let you understand your body's satiety levels a little better.

This is really easy to do and doesn't change what you eat at all. All you need to do is eat a meal with a good protein source like chicken, fish, steak, or even vegetable proteins like beans or tofu, and eat that part of the meal first. Don't go around the plate eating a little of everything, as it will cause your insulin levels to rise. Instead, eat all of your protein, THEN move on to everything else on your plate.

Eat Your Veggies and Fiber Next

This is not only going to help fill you up with the healthiest items on your plate, but it also helps to keep your insulin levels low. Every time your insulin levels rise, your body is going to stop burning fat for a certain period of time. You want to keep the levels as low as possible during your meals, which means saving all of the complex carbohydrates for last.

Once you have eaten your main protein source, you can then eat the salad or veggies on your plate, or any complex carbohydrates, like rice, quinoa, beans or lentils.

Save Refined Carbs for Last

Your carbs are going to be last, or in this case, the refined carbs. These will raise your glucose and insulin levels the fastest, plus they can cause you to overeat a bit. This is when you eat carbs like potatoes and bread. There is nothing wrong with eating a roll with dinner but try to save it for last.

HOW TO FOCUS ON BALANCE OF NUTRITION WHEN LOSING WEIGHT

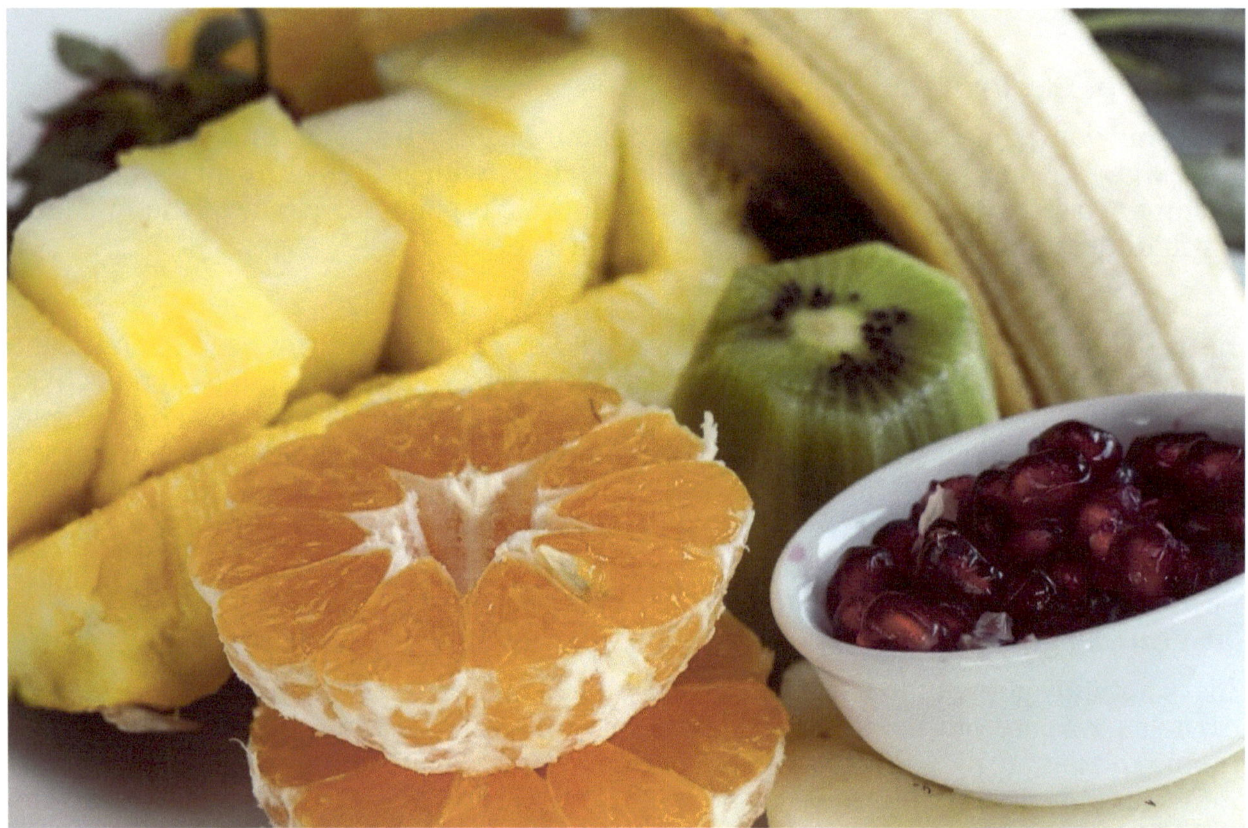

When you are working on losing a few extra pounds, it can be hard to figure out what to eat, or what not to eat. After all, weight loss is about 80% diet and 20% physical activity.

This means you should be focusing on what you are eating before anything else. The trick is to have a good balance of nutrients for every meal and snack, then stop eating when you're satiated. Here are some tips for keeping that balance.

Balancing Out Your Plate

The first thing to learn is how to find the right balance on your plate. This is going to vary a little depending on your own requirements, food intolerances and allergies, and personal preference. For example, if you are on a gluten-free diet, the carb section on your plate might be a little different than someone on a vegan diet where many of the foods they eat are low carbs.

However, here are some ways to balance out your plate so that you have all the nutrients you need with every meal and snack:

Protein, Carb, and Fat – The simplest way to create a balanced meal is to make sure you have at least one protein source, one carb, and one fat. This could be grilled salmon (protein and fat), brown rice (carb), and veggies (carb), or a big salad with chicken (protein), walnuts (fat), and veggies (carbs). There are many ways to use this type of balance for your meals.

Half Your Plate in Vegetables or Salad – This is another way to help make sure you get enough vegetables and fiber into your diet. This is when half your plate for lunch or dinner is a salad or vegetables, with the other half being split up into your protein and other food sources, such as carbs or fats.

80/20 Rule – This is good when you want a little treat with your meal, without going overboard. To balance it out, have 80 percent "healthy" food, with 20 percent being your "treat".

Healthy Foods for Each Nutrient

Another way to focus more on nutrition than diets when you are trying to lose weight is make a list of the most important nutrients you need, then find foods you enjoy for each of these nutrients. Here are some examples:

- Protein – Eggs, meat, poultry, fish, tofu, nuts, cheese/dairy, beans/legumes
- Carbs – brown rice, potatoes, quinoa, oats, most vegetables
- Fiber – Chia seeds, whole grains, brown rice, vegetables, fruits
- Fats – coconut oil, olive oil, avocado, nuts, fatty fish (salmon)

Stop with the All or Nothing Mentality

Through this balance of nutrition, you are going to stop dieting and restricting, and stop with the all or nothing mentality. There are no "bad" labeled foods, but instead you are going to just aim for a healthy balance between foods that nourish your body, and little treats that help to keep away those cravings.

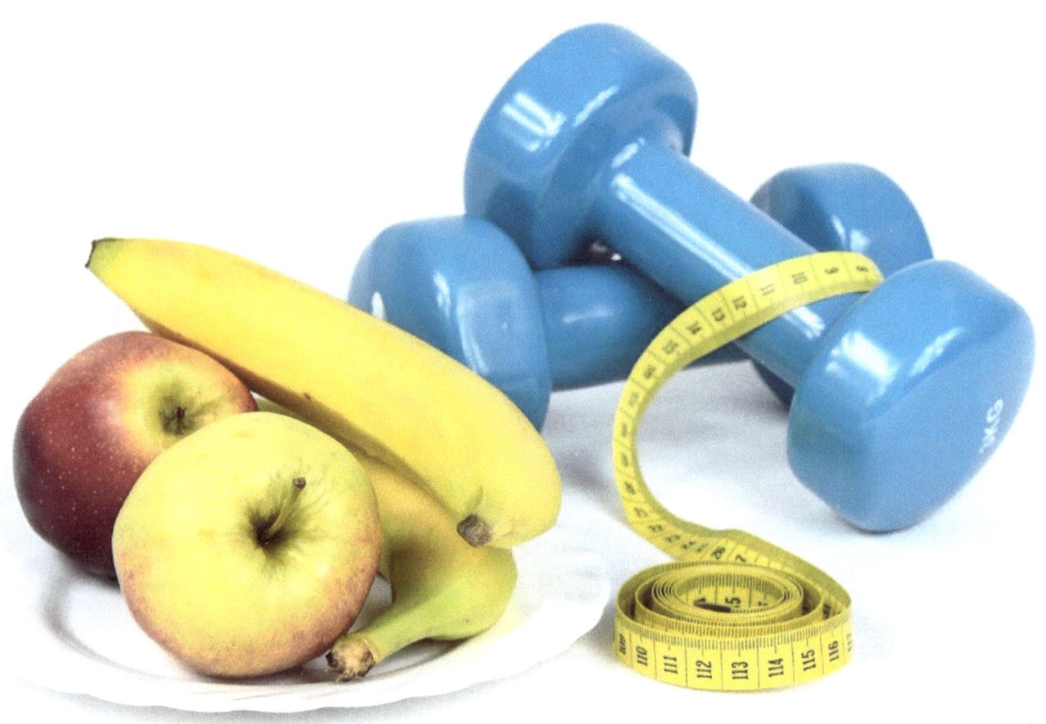

Weight loss can be among one of the most challenging projects to take on, but it can also be the most rewarding. There is a lot to be gained through learning how to control urges and habits; controlling eating habits is a major feat because of the availability and ease with which a person can use food to medicate themselves, but success can be just around the corner. In the next few paragraphs you'll learn about the biggest obstacles when trying to lose weight.

Attitude

You've probably heard some version of this a million times, but it's all about attitude. Your viewpoint can have a massive effect on the outcome, so it's important to have your mind in the right place when you're aiming to make such a huge change.

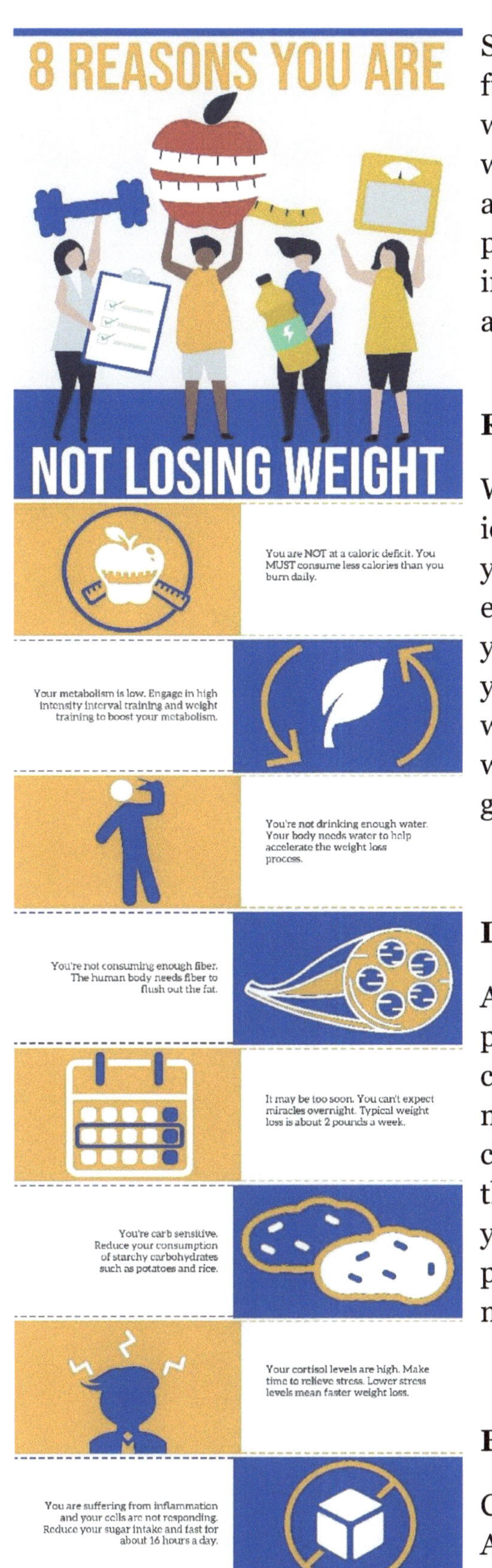

Some people view diets as a quick fix for some function or event, like a school reunion or upcoming wedding, but the most successful people who lose weight see it more as a lifestyle change that they have accepted. Losing focus can put an end to all the positive progress that you've discovered, so it's important to know what you're looking for, and make a decision.

Real Wellness

When you're making this kind of change, it's a good idea to do some serious soul searching. Try to look at your behaviors and how you deal with food. Pay especially close attention to the things that trigger your desire to eat. Knowing these things can protect you from a sudden urge that can come in without a warning during a weak moment. Caving into weakness will leave you feeling defeated, so it's a good idea to see what may come long beforehand.

Lifestyle

A lot of people seem surprised when they cut back on pizza, and go home to sit in front of the TV. Real change requires a good amount of effort, so you'll need to find out ways that you can begin to make changes to your lifestyle. That means getting up off the couch and taking a walk several times a week. If you're busy, you'll need to find a way to get that physical part of the work done. Even if it's just 15 minutes before your go to work each day.

Eating Habits

Changing how you eat is another part of the process. A lot of people use food replace feeling of belonging and other things. When you get a handle on your eating, it will have longer lasting effects on your weight and health.

One of the best things you can do is remove unhealthy foods from your kitchen and replace them with healthy fruits and veggies.

NUTRITION RED FLAGS TO WATCH OUT FOR

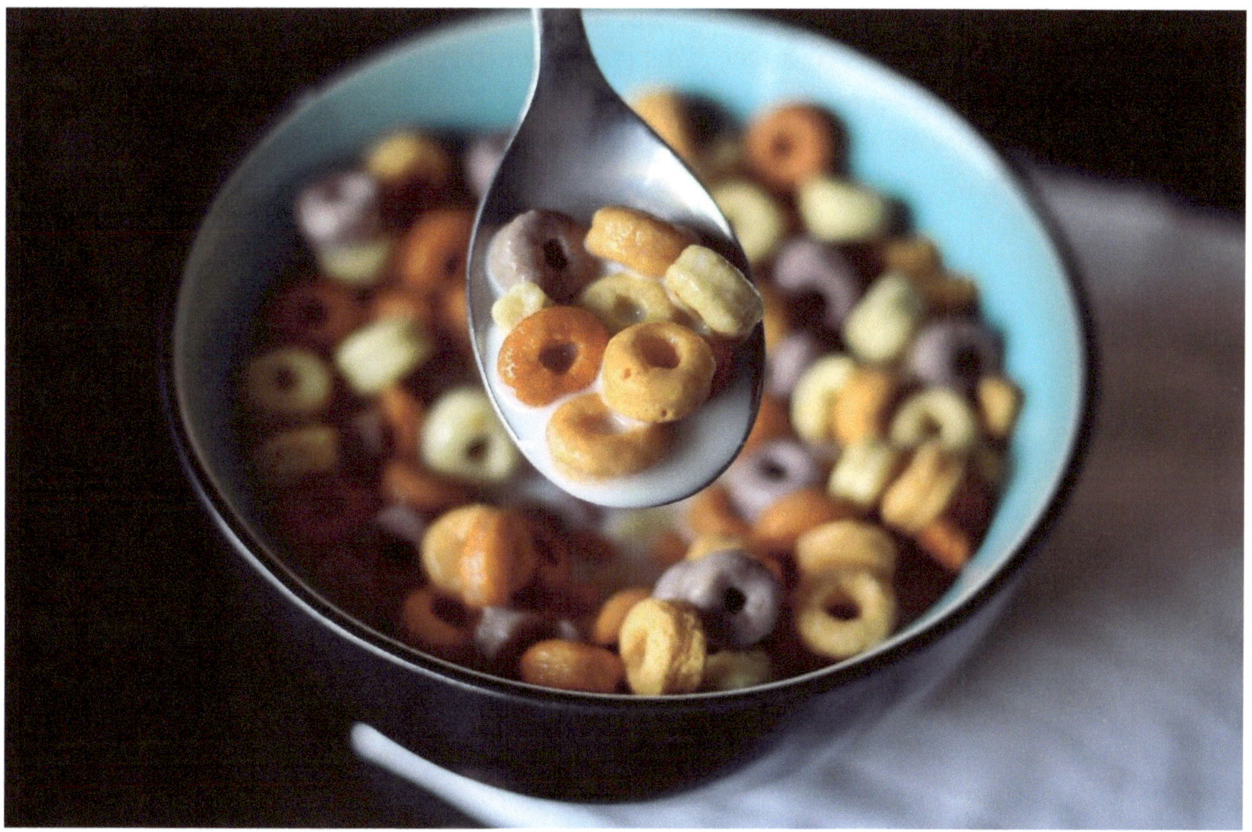

When you take a closer look at modern food production, you begin to notice that there are a lot of sneaky little things that companies can do to hide the facts about their products that more discerning consumers might want to know. These companies do whatever they can to hide negatively reviewed additives and preservatives of different types, so they might utilize tricks that can catch you off guard. In the next few paragraphs you'll find out what some of these tricks are and learn nutrition red flags to keep an eye out for.

Fiber Is Low or Missing Completely

This is one you will see a lot in the production of store-bought bread goods and snack cakes. Even though these foods once came from grains, the actual components of what made that food a grain are now gone, leaving only the gummy, flakey bots of what it used to be. When this fiber is removed, this gooey remnants of the food can stick to parts of your digestive tract and form pockets around areas in your intestines. These pockets can create serious issues down the road, years later. Processed grains also are a trigger for weight gain, so limiting your intake of these types of foods will be essential for health reasons.

Extra Sugars Are Added

Some foods have had a lot of things done to them to make sure that they can last in a truck that is traveling through the desert. Sometimes the processes can rob food of their flavor, so the next solution when it is a sweet food, is to simply add extra sugar. The sugar that was there is still there, only changed chemically, so now your body must deal with the sugar overload. This is especially bad for diabetic people. Sugars like these will appear as maltose, dextrose, high fructose corn syrup, and sucrose.

Trans Fats

This is a serious red flag. People really shouldn't eat any trans fats. They are very dangerous because they cause a reduction of healthy cholesterol and a rise in the bad cholesterol. For some people that could be deadly, and it's very bad for the heart. These foods are so bad that many companies have been ordered to stop using trans fats in the food production. There are a number of healthy snacks that you can have instead.

Talk about sneakiness. Look at the total fat content on a nutrition label. If the individual fat content does not add up to the total fat content, then the difference is trans fat. If the trans fat content is less than 1%, the FDA does not require that it be listed on the nutrition label. If you don't do the math, you would never know it is there.

During the 1980's, artificial sweeteners exploded into massive popularity. At the time, people were looking for alternative to sugar, which had been blamed for a lengthy laundry list of issues, and diabetes was one of the biggest. As the end of the 1990's approached, people began to make some evaluations about the legacy that these once celebrated magic powders was leaving for future generations, and it appeared that artificial sweeteners were no longer the hero of the story they previously had been. The purpose of the following article is to take a look at the role of sweeteners in health and weight loss.

Gathering the Data

What began as a few questions was soon a growing skepticism. Eventually, nearly 40 different studies were held to determine the effectiveness of these sweeteners. Not only did these sweeteners have to be effective as sweeteners, they were also tasked with being found worthy as effective weight loss management tools.

These studies looked at hundreds of thousands of people to test their reactions, collect observations, and measure individual progress. Each of these studies took place with the absolute adherence to procedure, and researchers were shocked to discover that many of the people in the trials who consumed the sweeteners were found to be at much higher risk for health issues like weight gain and heart disease than those who didn't.

What Happened?

This new information collected by the doctors had them confounded. At that point all that could be done was to begin testing new theories about why this weight gain, and diabetes had become associated with the sweeteners. Some possible explanations have questioned as to whether or not sweeteners could be causing some severe form of damage to the gut flora.

Still others believe it could be as simple as people rewarding themselves to extreme amounts while thinking that they haven't ingested as many calories. Either way, more testing will be needed to uncover exactly where things are going and what the status of sweeteners while in the future.

What Now?

A lot of people have begun to back away from sweeteners. Even many experts seem to have an aura of avoidance when it comes to these additives. When asked, many professionals will simply say that they don't believe that they are harmful in small amounts, but they believe that it probably would be better to limit how much a person has in general. The general consensus now is if you need a sweetener, go with real sugar. At least you know what is in it and that it came from natural sources instead of produced in a lab.

HOW MINDFUL EATING CAN HELP

Speaking of healthy weight loss and not sticking to diets, mindful eating can be effective at helping you to lose weight and keep it off. With mindful eating, you actually pay attention to the entire eating experience. It isn't about what you are eating, but HOW you are eating. You will be present during each meal, which really helps you to understand what nutrition you are feeding your body, and where to make changes.

How to Incorporate Mindful Eating into Your Routine

It can be really difficult to be mindful of your eating unless you decide to make a specific effort to do so. When you are used to one particular way of eating, and it has become a habit over the course of years as is common with most people, it's going to take more than just a few days to correct the behavior. In the next few paragraphs, you'll find a carefully crafted process that will show you how to incorporate mindful eating into your routine.

Increase Your Self Awareness

One thing that can be extremely jarring yet educational for your to do with yourself, is to try and gain more self-awareness for a few moments. When you're alone or isolated, you can gain habits that when revealed to the public, might seem odd to a few people.

This can be witnessed in poor eating habits like fast binge eating. In this practice, a person might shovel food into their mouth at such a rate that they don't even truly enjoy the food that they're eating and it's almost joyless. Try to notice how you feel before you begin to eat. Remember that it isn't a race, and that if you eat more slowly, you'll enjoy your food and feel more satisfied.

Take a Moment to Taste

Have you ever gotten a meal, only to discover that it's completely subpar, and you ate it just to get it over with? It's important to begin to draw distinctions between the meals that you enjoy and the meals that you are just eating out of boredom. You might be surprised that you don't really pay much attention to some meals, and that eating is just a formality to begin or end the day, or it is used as a comfort to combat a stressful situation. Taking an inventory of what you really feel will help you to make better choices, and you know that higher quality healthy foods will almost always taste a lot better.

Avoid the Tech Zombie Binge

It can be really dangerous to good eating habits to eat while you're reading things online or watching a good TV show. This can lead to eating out of control and you might end up finishing an entire bag of snacks that were meant to last a week. If you are less distracted, it's easier to control how much food you are eating. The time you spend with your food should be spent developing good habits that lay the path for better, more healthy choices in the future.

How Mindful Eating Works

Mindful eating works just like any other mindful practice you have. You are going to be completely present during your meal, appreciating every bite, paying attention to the experience, chew each bite slowly and most importantly, noticing how your body feels when you eat certain foods.

Most people eat very mindlessly. You might watch TV while eating chips out of a bag, or rush through dinner because you have plans afterward. This can cause you to get gas and bloating from eating too fast, eat the wrong foods for your body, and overeat.

With mindful eating, you are paying attention to your body and really reveling in each bite, which in turn can allow you to see what foods your body loves, and which aren't nourishing it much.

Using Mindful Eating to Lose Weight

The reason this helps you lose weight is all in your mentality and in the practice itself. Here are some reasons mindful eating can help you to lose weight:

- You don't overeat as much.
- You start figuring out what fuels your body.
- You understand more about nourishing your body with important nutrients.
- By changing the eating habit, you don't just snack all day long.
- You learn to listen to your body's cues.

Just give it a try! Sit quietly during your next meal, with no phone and no TV nearby. Focus on what you are eating, eat slowly and mindfully, and be present. You will notice just how amazing this experience can be.

EATING TO REDUCE INFLAMMATION

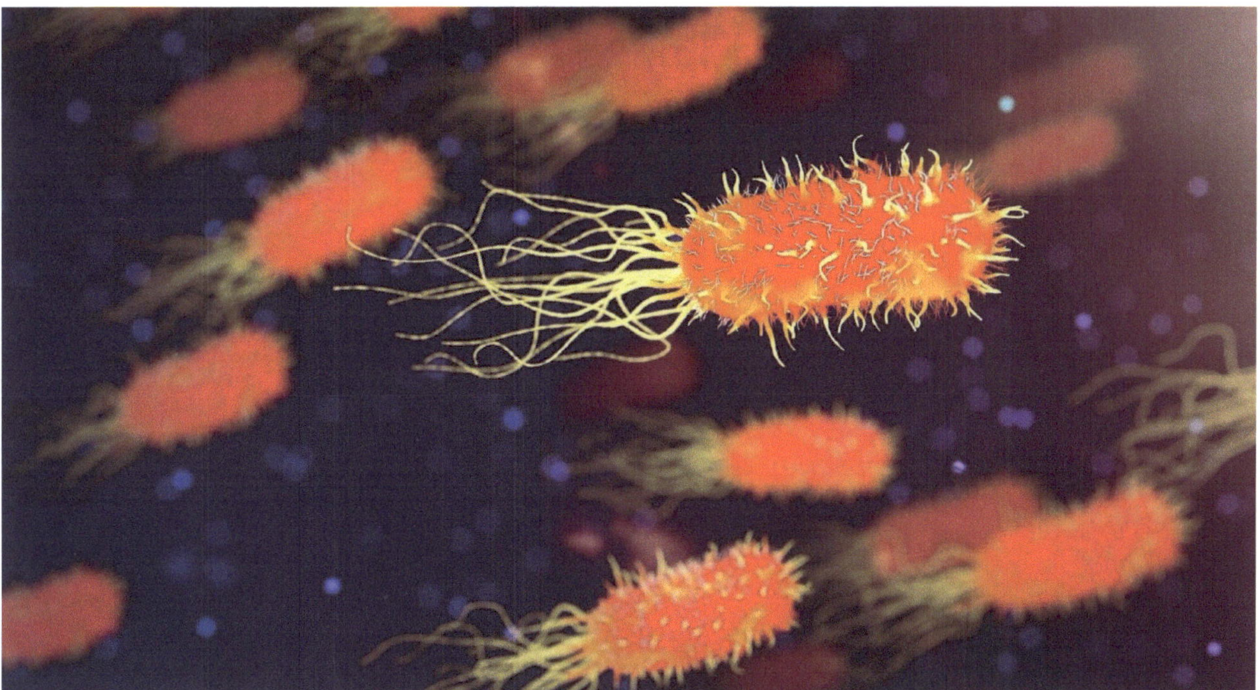

Do you have a problem with inflammation in your body? As people grow older, inflammation becomes a greater issue. Inflammation is also a major side effect and cause of sustained injuries and discomfort. What you might not know is that there are ways to get some relief that are inexpensive options. If you've been hoping to find ways to aid your body in the search for relief without getting into a whole new culture dominated by medications of various types, then you might want to review the next few paragraphs on eating to reduce inflammation.

Limit Your Intake of Acidic Foods

It's no secret that people love their bacon and eggs, but you need to be careful about how much of these kinds of foods that you eat. Acidic foods can put a lot of strain on your system, and they can be devastating when you are having issues with inflammation. It's best to avoid processed and refined sugars, bleached flours and dairy foods during flare up periods. Remember, you don't have to quit forever, just as long as you need to deal with the inflammation.

Eat Lots of Deep Greens

One thing that you can remember that will help you is that the deep green vegetables are usually the ones that you want to eat when you're having issues with inflammation. Celery is also a powerful anti-inflammatory, so you can get a lot of its benefits by simply drinking a cup of soup broth with a lot of celery in it. Cucumber, spinach, and kale are among some of the other most beneficial veggies in this group, and almost all of them make great side dishes for any meal.

On a side note, there are also tons of fruits that can do a similar job, just be sure that they are alkalizing like papaya.

Get in A Good Workout

If you need a more active way to combat this acidity, then a good 30 to 40-minute workout will definitely do the trick. Sweating is another really great way that your body uses to get rid of excess acids and wastes. If you can get some good exercise in, you'll pump more blood and oxygenate it so that it can feed your muscles more easily. You'll also increase your blood alkalinity and burn extra calories in the process.

Cut Back on Drinking

Most alcoholic drinks are filled with sugar. As you've seen before, sugars in drinks and foods can be highly acidic, so naturally, the less you have of these, the healthier you will likely feel. Alcohol also keeps your body from metabolizing anything other than sugar, so it could have a range of side effects that you would rather skip.

WHAT IS INTUITIVE EATING?

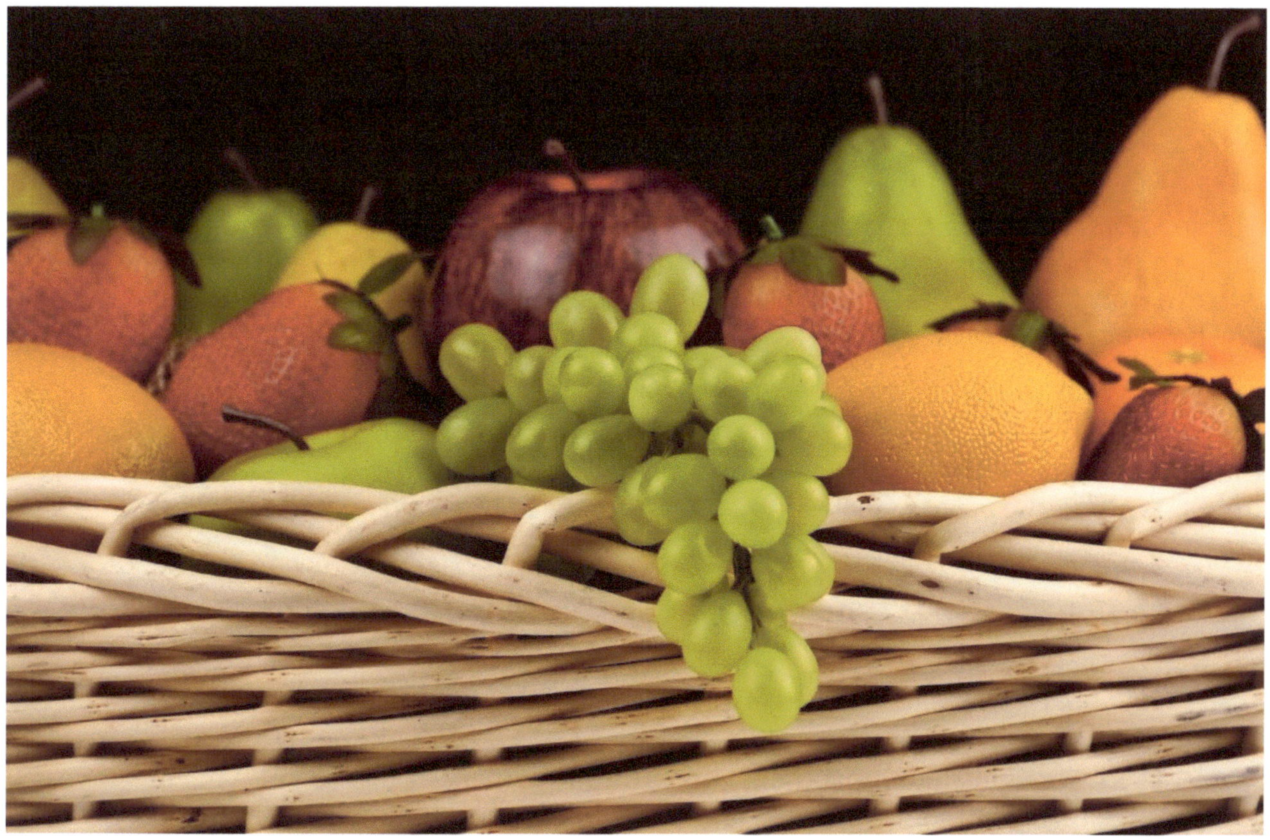

The next part of healthy weight loss has to do with intuitive eating, which can also be combined with mindful eating.

What is intuitive eating? This is where you learn to listen to your body to decide what to eat and how much. Nothing is off the table, there are no restrictions, and there is no calorie counting, carb counting, or specific diets.

It does take some practice, but when you learn how to give your body what it needs, you naturally lose weight and get to a good mental place at the same time.

Listening to Your Body

You will first need to learn how to listen to your body, which is the most important part of intuitive eating, but also the most difficult. People who are going from yo-yo diets to this way of eating find many challenges. You fear gaining back all the weight you lost, and struggle with suddenly being allowed to eat whatever you want without guilt or regret.

The most important thing to remember is this – everything will even out and level out in time. In the beginning, you just focus on eating whatever you crave, not worrying about what or how much you eat. This is to heal your relationship with food and stop putting levels on everything.

Then you go through other stages of eating, like listening to your body, understanding the difference between satiety and being full, coming to terms with the feeling of hunger, understanding the hunger scale, and trying to figure out exactly what your body is craving.

It Doesn't Happen Overnight

This is not a quick fix and you won't start losing weight immediately. In fact, it can take longer to lose weight than most diets and workout plans, but you are looking at longevity here. You are healing your relationship with food, nourishing your body, and getting rid of that diet mentality.

What you need is patience, kindness, and the understanding that you will be healing your body from the inside out.

Reaching Your Body's Natural Weight

Another thing to understand about intuitive eating is that it's not about losing the most weight or being a certain size. When you follow it correctly, listen to your body, and eat whatever your body needs at the time, you will eventually reach your body's natural weight. The weight and size it is meant to be, not the size you always wanted to be.

Remember a goal should be attainable. You will never be a size 2 if your body was meant to be a size 8. It just won't happen. Get to the weight you were meant to be and be happy at that weight.

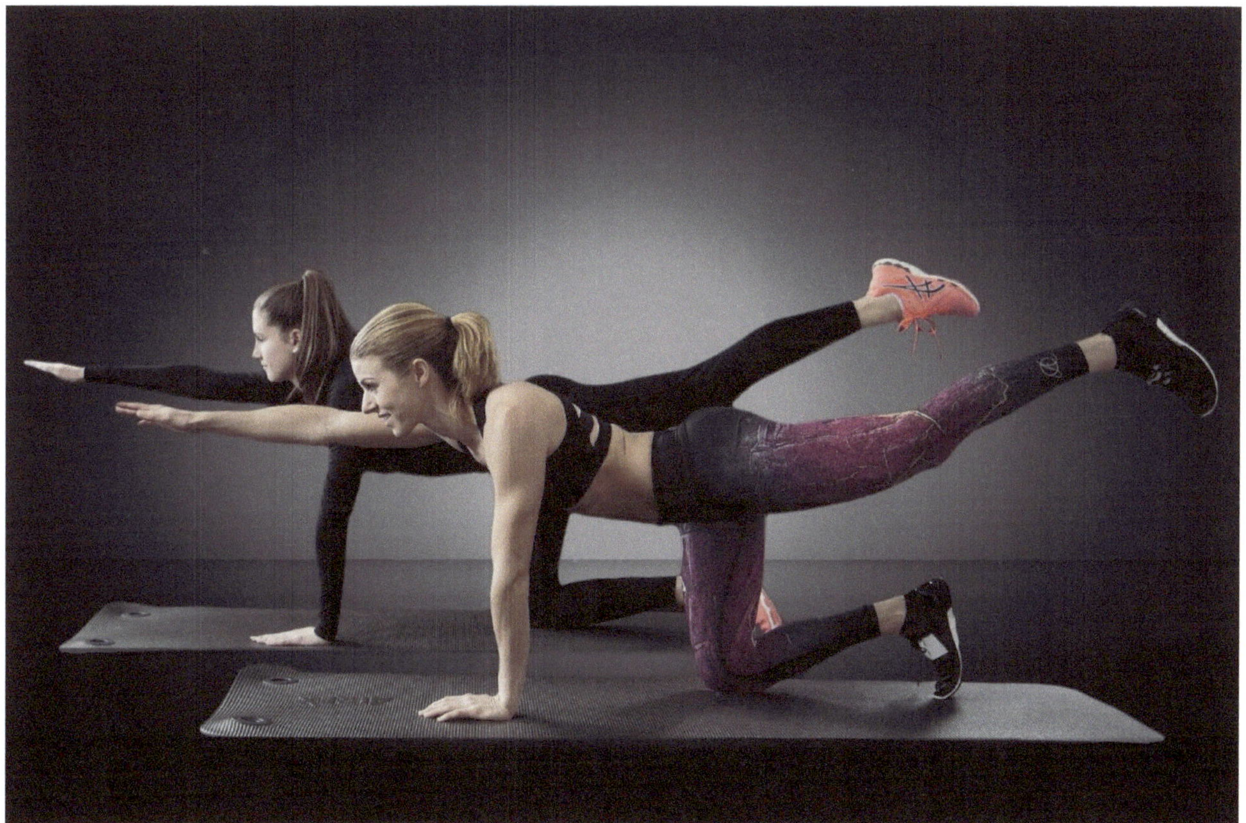

After you have figured out the diet aspect of your weight loss efforts, it is time to move on to fitness. This, as you know, makes up about 20% of your weight loss journey.

The problem isn't starting a fitness program for most people but keeping up with it. Here are some tips for finding what will motivate you to stick with it.

Changing Your Mindset About Fitness

While you are changing how you think about food and diets, you also want to change your mindset around exercise. Instead of thinking about it just for weight loss, think about it for your health. Get it into your head that you are working out for your health, including mental and physical health.

Remind yourself that it is good for your heart, it improves your strength and flexibility, it is wonderful for joint pain, it will help manage stress and reduce anxiety. There are many reasons to exercise aside from just losing or maintaining your weight, though those are definite bonuses of it.

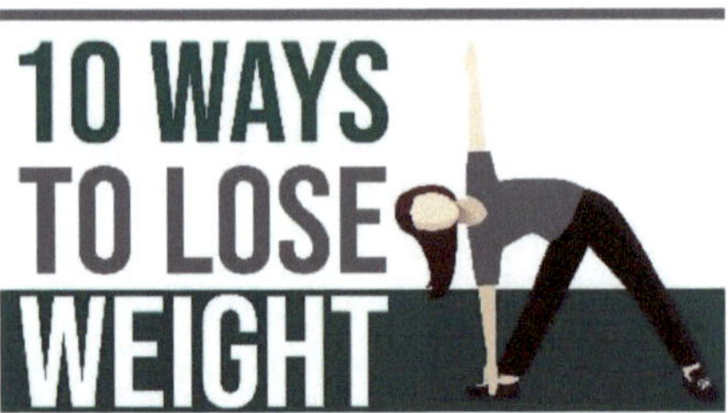

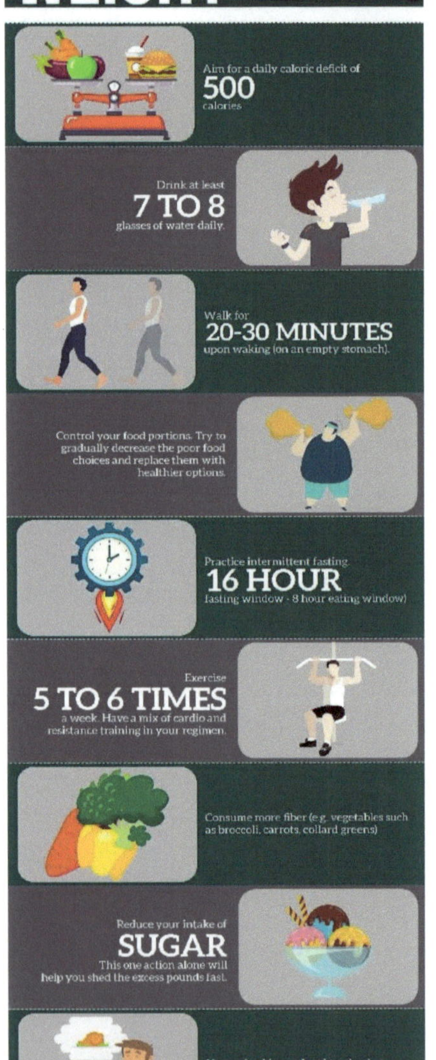

Find Exercises You Love

You also want to have fun with your fitness routine, which means finding exercises you love to do. Even if you have always imagined exercise to be a chore, there is something out there for you, you just have to find it.

Experiment, try different classes, check out local boutique gyms in your area, think about something you have always wanted to do. Here are some options that go beyond the standard exercises:

- Indoor rock climbing
- Tai chi
- Yoga or Pilates
- Dance classes
- Biking

Stop Feeling Forced to Exercise

You don't want to feel like you are forced to exercise, otherwise it will keep feeling like a chore, and eventually you will give up. Change your entire mindset around fitness. Think of it as something that is great for your body, will give you energy, and will help with your mental health and wellness, and fun to do.

With these simple changes, you can start working on improving your overall health and well-being. You will suddenly have less stress, stronger muscles, and yes, less weight on your body, which helps with joint pain.

You want to develop daily healthy habits, from drinking more water and fueling your body with healthy foods, to making sure you get regular physical activity. This is what will make a difference – this is who you will lose weight this year and actually keep it off.

UNDERSTANDING THE LATEST FITNESS BOOM

Health in general has gotten even more popular recently, but so has fitness. Everywhere you look, people are buying workout apparel, posting their workouts on social media, and signing up for 5k and 10k races. Why is that? Here is a look at where the most recent trend in fitness is coming from.

There is a Bigger Focus on Health

The good news is a big part of the reason for the latest fitness trend boom is that everyone wants to be healthier. There seems to be a bigger focus on health, as opposed to being a certain size or sticking to a trendy diet. This is great! It means more people are working out for their overall health, not just for weight loss.

People Love Signing Up for Races

You have probably seen pictures of your friends or co-workers running a race, such as a 5k, 10k, or a themed race like the Bubble Run or the Color Run. These are a lot of fun to participate in, not to mention how great they are for fitness, and for whichever charity they are helping to fund. This makes it to where a lot more people are training for the races at the gym, on the treadmill at home, or with groups on the street.

There are Budget-Friendly Gyms

It used to be that signing up for a gym membership was the most expensive way to get fit and lose weight, but that couldn't be further from the truth nowadays. Many gyms are popping up in cities and towns that are around $10 a month, allowing you to work out for much less than if you had to buy workout DVDs or equipment at home.

Boutique-Style Gyms are all the Rage

Another type of gym that is becoming a trend and leading to the fitness craze is the boutique-style gym. Instead of a gym with exercise rooms and tons of equipment, these gyms are usually for one specific purpose. There are CrossFit gyms, women-only gyms, indoor trampoline gyms, Pilates gyms, and many more. They are much smaller and intended to fit less people at one time, often structured in classes or with personal trainers helping just a few people at a time.

Social Media Influence

Finally, people love sharing about their workouts online! Much of the fitness craze is from other sharing what they're doing on Facebook, Instagram, and Twitter. You get inspiration from others, and you can motivate your friends by showing what workouts you're doing.

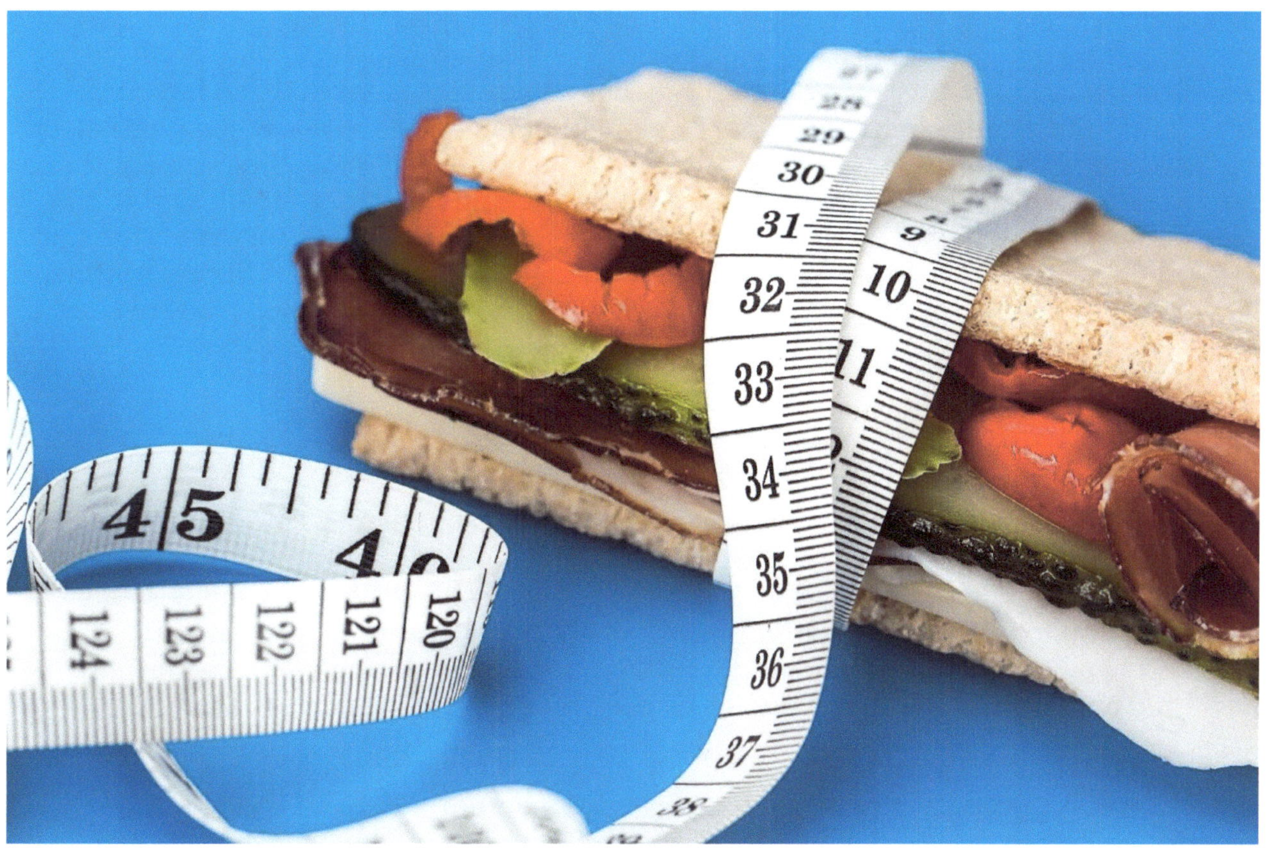

If you have set a New Year's resolution of losing weight, you might be a little lost with how to begin. Here are some helpful tips:

Setting Your Weight Loss Goals

Before you get started with your weight loss New Year's resolution, you need to have some goals in mind. It is important that you try to be realistic with your goals, and instead of just saying you want to lose X number of pounds, you have some actionable goals as well. For each health or weight loss goal you set for yourself as your resolution, list some actions that you should do in order to achieve those goals.

Setting Actionable Goals

An actionable goal is one where you can define exactly what needs to be done to achieve it. If you want to fly a plane someday, the actions would be to learn how to fly planes and get your private pilot's license. The same concept works with any type of weight loss goals you have.

You need to start by choosing a realistic goal for your New Year's weight loss, whether that means losing a certain amount of weight in the year or losing 1-2 pounds a week consistently. You might also decide to choose a goal based on the size of clothing you wear.

Once you have chosen the realistic goal, you will then need to make a list of actionable steps it takes to achieve that larger goal. This might help you choose smaller goals along the way as well. If you want to lose 50 pounds by the end of the year, then you know you need to lose about 4 pounds a month. This is just 1 pound a week, so it falls within the reasonable goal category. Now decide how you can lose a pound a week, from what diet you should follow, to healthy lifestyle changes to make, like following a fitness routine, cutting out sugar, or stopping late-night snacking. This gives you a good place to start with your New Year's resolution.

SCHEDULING EXERCISE INTO YOUR DAILY SCHEDULE

One of the problems with starting a new fitness routine isn't having the motivation to do it in the beginning of the year but making it a part of your new lifestyle. A New Year's resolution shouldn't just be something you do for the first few weeks of January but encourage you to make a brand-new lifestyle change. It is meant to turn you into a stronger, healthier, and fitter person overall. This means choosing a fitness routine, switching it up as needed, and really making it a part of your regular schedule.

By including it in your schedule just like any other appointment, you are going to keep up with it a lot better and treat it just as important as your weekly nail appointment or going to the dentist. Here are some more tips for keeping up with your fitness routine:

Turn it Into a Fun Challenge With Friends

Making new lifestyle changes and doing it all on your own can be a huge bummer. It also keeps you from really answering to someone and motivating yourself to exercise on days when you would really rather skip the gym. A good way to keep up with it on a regular basis is to start a challenge with your friends. Put together a group of friends that will keep each other motivated, where you check in, and maybe even offer a prize to the person who walks the most steps or runs the most miles in a certain period of time. The challenge keeps everyone in the group accountable for the new weight loss goals you have, and you can even get together to work out together if you all live local.

Think About it More as a Healthy Lifestyle Change

Sometimes, weight loss and working out is all about your mindset. Don't just think about it as a short-term goal, but as a brand-new lifestyle change. Think about yourself in a year, 10 years, or 20 years, and see how you will still be working out. You may be leaner and fitter, but you will still be dedicated to being healthy and fit. You want this to be something you do for the good of yourself and for your family. Perhaps you have young kids and you want to be a good role model for them. Working out regularly is something they will see you doing, which can help battle childhood obesity.

Make Sure You Are Doing It For the Right Reasons

One of the things that often leads to failure is losing weight or working out for the wrong reasons. If you are doing it to impress someone or because your significant other has made comments, you are not doing it for the right reasons. This is not going to be enough to see it through and gives you an unhealthy mindset from the very beginning. However, once you have made the decision for yourself because you want to be healthier, then you will notice it is a lot easier to motivate yourself to exercise every day.

Have a Good Workout Area

If you intend to do most of your working out at home, then make sure you have a dedicated area. This keeps you from getting distracted and becomes your quiet space where you focus on your fitness routine. This can be a treadmill in your bedroom, elliptical machine and trampoline in your family room, or an office you are converting to a home gym. Just be consistent and try to exercise in the same place each time.

TOOLS FOR TRACKING YOUR WEIGHT LOSS

Another thing to get ready before the New Year arrives is to have a tool for tracking your weight loss. You don't need to spend a lot of money or have a fancy tool either; it can be as simple as using pen and paper. Just decide on the method that will work best for you. Here are some options for tracking your weight loss:

Get a Digital Scale

If you are more concerned about pounds on the scale than your measurements, then getting a digital scale is highly recommended. This keeps you from guessing what pound you are at, such as with a regular weight scale. The numbers are right there, and many newer ones also have some advanced features.

Make sure you use the scale at the same time of the day each time, with the same clothing. If you choose to weigh yourself Monday mornings at 6:00am with no clothes on, then try to be consistent each time you weigh yourself on the scale.

Use Pen and Paper

While many people like to use apps on their phone for tracking weight loss, you can just use a pen and paper. If you are using a journal to log your food and exercise, that same journal can be a wonderful tool for tracking your weight as well. Every time you weigh yourself or take measurements, jot it down in your journal to keep track of your progress.

HOW A BULLET JOURNAL CAN HELP YOU LOSE WEIGHT

If you are trying to lose weight but struggling to set the right goals or keep up with your daily motivation, using a bullet journal can definitely help. This allows you to know what to focus on, take a healthier approach to weight loss, and have a way to check in regularly so you keep up with your weight loss motivation.

Keep reading to learn how using a bullet journal can actually help you lose weight.

You Can Set Goals

The first way bullet journals help you to lose weight is by helping you set goals. You might set goals in a regular journal, but that is hard to keep track of because that same journal might be used for other things as well. With a bullet journal, you have a page or section dedicated to your weight loss, tend to use it more often, and have a really handy way to set multiple goals and reward yourself when you reach them.

You can set all types of goals related to your health and weight loss, like how many pounds you want to lose, ideal measurements, clothing sizes to fit into, healthy foods to eat, diet plans to follow, fitness goals, water goals, and so much more. The options really are customized to you and what your personal goals are.

There is a Place to 'Check In'

The great thing about bullet journaling is that you probably use it daily or close to that, which gives you an easy way to check in with your progress. You can track your weight and measurements, write down what you ate that day or record how much water you drank. Checking in is a way to be accountable for yourself and your own goals, which is really important if you need accountability that is more private.

Meal Planning

The bullet journal can also be the perfect place for planning out your meals. This works for any type of diet you are following, intuitive eating, and just trying to eat a healthier diet overall. You can write down what meals you want to have each week, decide on a meal prepping day, write to-do lists for shopping and preparing, and anything else you feel will be important for you to keep track of.

Plus, when using future weeks' meal planning, you can look back on the older pages and see what meals you tried that you liked. Now you know which ones to have weekly, and which ones you didn't really enjoy that much.

Other Ways to Track Your Health

Don't forget you can track anything with your health, not just weight lost. The bullet journal is a great way to make sure you drink enough water, get regular exercise, have doctor check-ups, and take your medication as prescribed.

Download an App

Apps are good for convenience and to easily enter your weight or measurements. They are also good because you get graphs of how much you have lost over a certain period of time. Some apps, such as MyFitnessPal, will also provide other resources, such as tracking your fitness, food, and water intake each day.

Keep a Spreadsheet

If you like to use your computer for tracking weight loss, consider starting an Excel spreadsheet or use whatever spreadsheet program you prefer. Enter the date and the weight or measurements in whatever increments you prefer, then leave a space for any notes you find relevant.

Take Your Measurements

Taking your measurements is another good way to keep track of your weight loss. Before the New Year begins, get a flexible measuring tape like the ones fabric stores and craft supply stores have for sewing. Measure around your upper arms, thighs, waist, hips, breasts, and buttocks for accurate measuring. Write down or record the measurements in whatever tool you have decided to use. This is often good because muscle weighs more than fat, so if you are doing a lot of weight training, you can better see your body changing through measurements.

Consider Your Clothing Size

Another way to see how much weight you have been losing is to consider your clothing size. You might notice that even if the scale doesn't reflect your weight loss, your jeans are suddenly loose, or you can fit into your 'skinny clothes'. Put on some of your smaller sized clothes throughout the year to track your progress.

Because muscle weighs more than fat, you might not see the number on the scale change or it might even go up as you build muscle, but you will see the difference in how your clothes fit because you have lost inches instead of pounds.

FOCUSING ON A BALANCE BETWEEN NUTRITION AND FITNESS

Now that you know what your goals are, it is time to delve into those actionable diet and fitness steps. You probably know by now that both diet and exercise are equally important when you are trying to lose weight. If you only change your diet, but continue living a sedentary lifestyle, you might lose a little weight, but it is hard to keep up the same level of weight loss throughout the year. You need a good way to burn off excess calories, which means adding in exercise. Plus, fitness is important for general health, just like changing your eating habits.

You also don't want to just workout more but continue eating whatever you want. There needs to be a balance between the two. You don't need to exercise 2 hours a day, 7 days a week and follow a 1,000-calorie diet every day either; in fact, these are unhealthy habits to start. Here are some tips for finding a good balance between improving both your nutrition and fitness:

Start exercising slowly – To start with your workout routine, start exercising slowly. This is especially important if you are accustomed to a sedentary lifestyle but want to begin working out more in the new year. You should not just start with marathon training right away or begin running 10 miles from the very first day. Regardless of the type of exercise routine you intend to begin, do it slowly and gradually. Work up to your ultimate fitness goals.

Choose a fitness routine you will enjoy – It is also important that you choose an exercise you are going to enjoy doing. It might seem great that you can walk every day, but if you hate walking, you won't keep up with it. One idea is to switch to a more enjoyable form of walking, such as hiking or walking by the beach. On the other hand, you can choose another exercise entirely, such as yoga, kick boxing, swimming, or playing a sport like tennis. There are lots of ways to get in your daily exercise to help you lose weight.

Know how many calories exercises will burn – Speaking of the balance between nutrition and fitness, part of the reason you exercise to lose weight is to burn more calories. This means knowing exactly how many calories to burn, and what exercises burn the most calories. If you are using cardio machines, such as elliptical trainers or treadmills, the machines will let you know how many calories you have burned. For other exercises, you should use a fitness tracker.

Calculate how many calories you need to eat daily – Make sure with your nutrition, you know what you are eating and how many calories you are consuming. Even if you aren't following a low-calorie diet, this is a good way to know where you are at and track how much you eat each day. Eventually, you won't keep tracking your food, but it is good in the beginning.

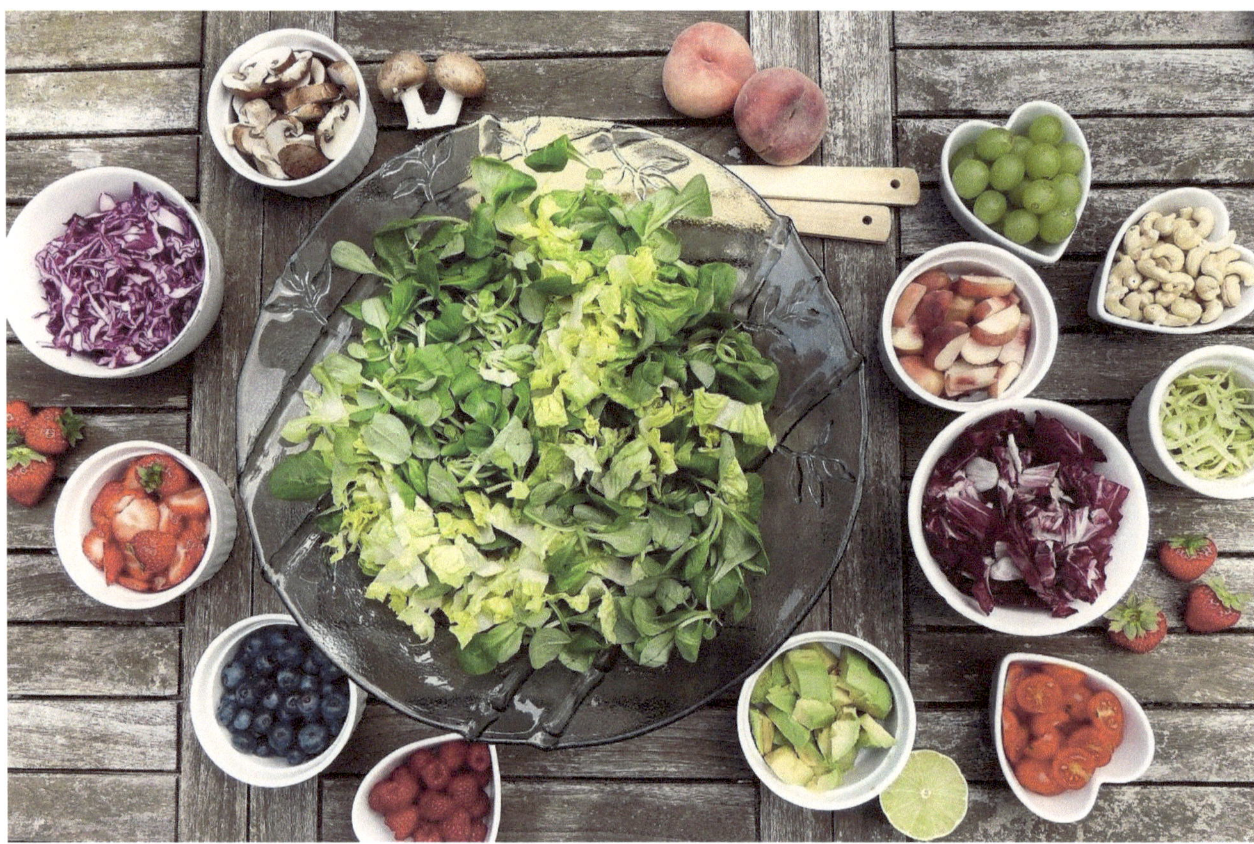

By this point, you are probably thinking about the different diets you can follow. Using the word 'diet' has negative connotation, making you feel like you are depriving yourself of something, so it is important to first get into the proper mindset. Look at it to change your dietary habits, not necessarily following a restricting diet; think healthy eating plan instead of diet.

There are a lot of different diets you can follow, depending on your needs and what your food preferences are. If you are a vegetarian currently, you might not like a diet like Paleo where it relies heavily on meat. You can still be a vegetarian Paleo, but it is difficult and not the best option when you are first starting out. Before the New Year arrives, it is good to decide what you will eat or what diet you will follow. Learn a little about each one until one really strikes you as something you can do.

Here are some options:

- Paleo

- [Keto](#)
- Whole30 or [Whole Foods Diet](#)
- Low-Fat or [Low-Calorie](#)
- [Vegetarian](#) or Vegan
- Raw Foods
- [Mindful](#)
- [Mediterranean](#)
- Or from these [12 diets](#)

The diets listed here are not necessarily "fad diets", but ones that do rely heavily on switching to a healthier lifestyle. Make sure you have done your research and look at what you can or can't eat in each diet so you can decide on the best one. This can really help you to decide which one is going to be the best option for you. Don't feel like you need to choose something because it is popular or because your friends are doing it.

Also, don't feel restricted to follow all the rules of the diet you choose. You can create your own custom diet as long as you are eating healthier, watching your portion sizes, and trying to consume as many vitamins and minerals as possible.

It is also recommended that you talk to your doctor or a nutritionist before making major changes to your diet.

WHY SWITCH TO A PLANT-BASED DIET?

As the conditions of meat production and the general public perception of meats have become larger and louder questions asked around the world, [plant-based diets](#) have had somewhat of a sudden surge in popularity. Great access to foods and information has made [plant-based diets](#) more accessible to larger groups of people, but you might be wondering why anyone would want to make that switch to a plant-based diet? If you continue reading the following article, you might find some reasons that will interest you.

High Fiber

Plant-based diets tend to be high fiber. The most important function of fiber is that it helps to keep your intestines clean. This is a big deal for you because cleans intestines will help you to absorb your food properly. This cuts back on buildup of methane gases that are produced in the intestines. These gases can gather quite quickly if your body doesn't make a clean sweep sometime in a day or two. This can cause discomfort and make riding with you in an enclosed space a regrettable experience.

You'll Lose Weight

People who eat primarily vegetable sources of food tend to be leaner. This is likely because they consume less of the undesired saturated fats that are connected with animal fats. Choosing more plant-based foods over animal-based foods will also see healthier numbers because they tend to be filling with a lot less sugars and calories. Because many of the foods you will be eating are whole and not processed, your body will be more apt to gain the nutrients that might have been blocked from absorption by chemicals used in preserving processed meats.

Heart Disease

It should be no surprise that people with a mainly plant-based diet experience lower numbers of heart disease. The most common factor for the healthier groups was simply that they ate a lot more fruits and vegetables than the groups with higher heart disease rates. Not only where there less heart attacks, but also less strokes and other heart related illness.

Healthy Skin

Few people realize that saturated fats can actually affect the skin. When the body is eliminating fats from the body, pores can become clogged with these fats and become deposits on the skin. When you eat more fruits and vegetables instead, then the various chemicals like lycopene work to aid all sorts of different systems within your body. These little nutrients can help your body to fight various types in infection and can even kill early formations of cancer cells in your body.

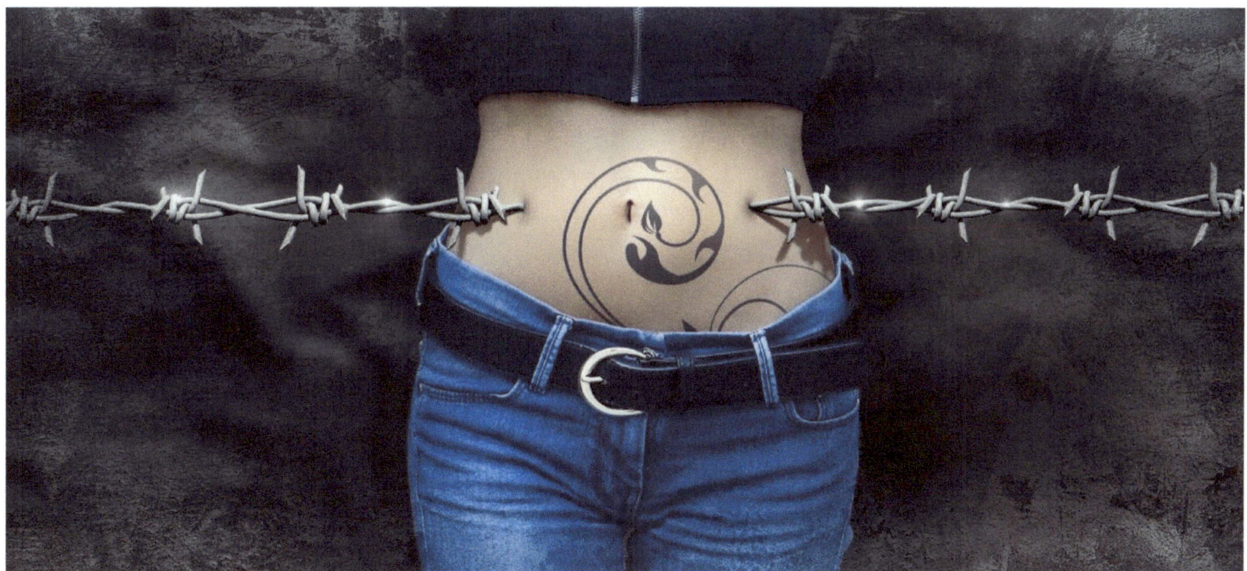

How well do you listen to your body when it has something to tell you? If you're like most people, then you probably feel like you're relatively in touch with your body and how it feels and functions from one day to the next, but it's easy to overlook certain signs that your body may be putting out to tell you something. To find out if this is happening to you, then it's probably a good idea to look at the kinds of things that happen to you when you need to find out what your gut might be telling you.

Your Stomach Gets Upset

How often do you suddenly get a serious bout with gas and bloating? When your bowel regularity changes, and you begin to experience all sorts of problems like diarrhea and constipation, then that could be a serious sign that something is very wrong in your gut. When your gut is healthy, then things should basically function smoothly and without a lot of fanfare.

Some further investigation is likely needed, so it's always good to go through a process of elimination when trying to find answers.

Sudden Food Intolerances

As you go through life, the content of your gut flora will change, but it would be highly unusual for you to suddenly be unable to eat specific foods. This kind of situation is most often the result in the degradation of gut flora in your body. Making sure that they are healthy and reproducing properly will help your gut to be able to process the foods that you eat more efficiently. When things begin to fail, diarrhea, bloating, gas, and pain will all become apparent. When this is the case, you might need to employ the use of specific life cultures in food to balance your gut flora properly.

Sudden Weight Gain or Loss

This is almost always a sign of gut flora issues. Weight gain that takes place without a change in habits is a sign that your body isn't processing the foods that you eat efficiently. When you gut isn't balanced properly, you will lose some of your ability to absorb nutrients, will results in fat storage and thus weight gain.

Constant Tiredness

When your stomach isn't working properly, it can mess up lots of different process, including those that control how well you can sleep at night. Over time, this fatigue can become constant. This can be helped by making sure that your gut contains colonies of healthy gut flora that you need to break down the food you eat.

THE QUALITY OF YOUR FOOD MATTERS

How important is the quality of food to you? Some people have the viewpoint that it doesn't really what they eat, and that it doesn't really matter where it comes from, but is that really true? Food is grown and manufactured all over the world, but not all companies and methods are created on an equal quality base. You might be really unhappy with one method versus another, so in the interest of spreading some important information, the next few paragraphs will be dedicated to explaining why the quality of your food matters.

Food Safety

One of the primary things that can create a steep divide between what is eaten in one culture versus another might be food safety standards. These standards have been created, reviewed and put into place to provide safety and reliability for consumers that they can have some belief in when making choices. There are nations and areas that don't adhere to these standards, and so there may be more instances of foodborne illness that are acceptable in one area compared to another. Some countries may produce goods that appear to be safe for using in cooking, but if they don't have the same standards as other developed nations, then dangerous metals might find their way into your food.

Nutrition

Food that is fresh is the most nutritious. If a company mass produces foods that will have to travel a long way, then the food is more than likely to have lost a large portion of its nutrients in whatever processes that have been employed to extend the shelf life of the product. Without the proper presence of nutrition, the food you ingest becomes empty calories that can cause people to gain weight while still craving nutrients their body needs causing them to overeat. Good quality foods will satisfy you properly instead of leaving you feeling like you haven't eaten anything. Whole foods are always the best option when they're available.

Processing Methods

Some of the processing methods used by companies require them to use chemicals that are often less than favorable. These can also include preservatives that help rob the food of their original flavor that has to be replaced by other artificial substances. Prepackaged foods are also astronomically high in sodium. Most foods that are frozen like gas station burritos are likely to contain 4 - 6 times the sodium you should have in day, only in just one or two serving sizes. Try to stick to the foods that you can cook for yourself with whole ingredients. It will be healthier and you'll know what in it. If you're in a serious time crunch, then there are some frozen meals made with health in view.

WAYS TO USE APPLE CIDER VINEGAR IN YOUR DIET

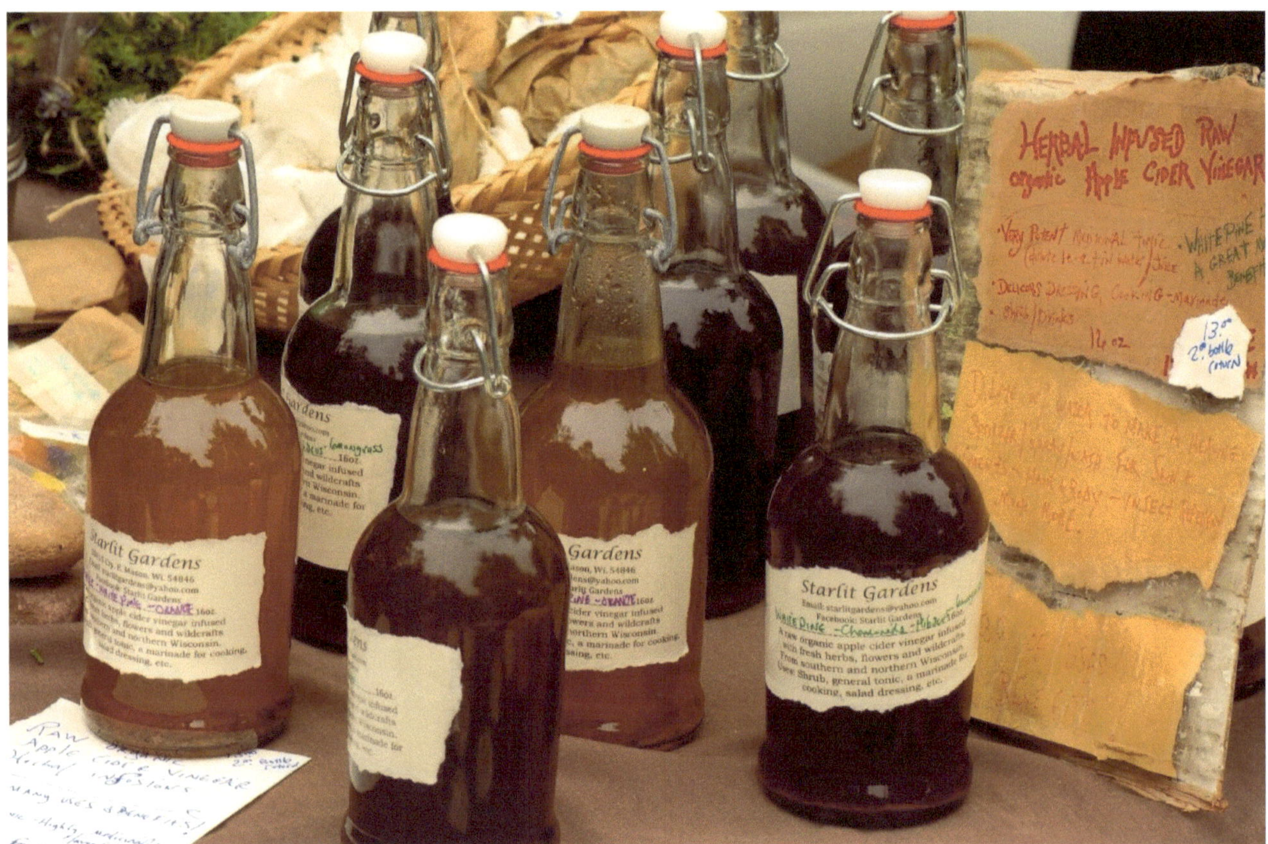

If you've been reading up on the great things that apple cider vinegar can do for you, then you probably heard that it can have some positive effects on your diet as well. Apple cider vinegar has been used in all sorts of health tonics dating back to the 1800's. Although the mechanisms still aren't entirely understood, science has been able to observe a few of its positive effects. In the following article you'll find a few ways to use apple cider vinegar in your diet.

Blood Sugar Regulation

One of the most reported ways in which apple cider vinegar can be used if for blood sugar regulation. Studies were able to detect that people who had ingested apple cider vinegar with meals didn't show blood spikes as high as the people who hadn't ingested any. This means that having apple cider vinegar with food can be extremely beneficial for people with type 2 diabetes.

Helps Cholesterol Levels

Tests run by researchers have also shown that ingesting apple cider vinegar helps the body to break down cholesterol in the blood. The implication here are massive in that even if apple cider vinegar only worked in a very small way, the benefits would make a worthwhile part of any dietary regimen. For the best effect, it should probably be consumed in a very dilute form on an empty stomach first thing in the morning.

Antibacterial Agent

The acidity of apple cider vinegar proves to be a generally inhospitable environment for microbes of the invasive type. Apple cider vinegar can even be used to clean your food before you eat it, as well as flavor it. You can easily drizzle some over your salad to make sure that you're protected by some forms of bacteria that can live in lettuce, like e coli, while giving your greens that tangy flavor that you've been looking for.

As an Appetite Suppressant

People in studies involving apple cider vinegar had less of an appetite than those in the groups that hadn't had any. Scientists found that the result of the lowered blood sugar decreased the appetite, but researchers didn't feel like this secondary effect was as important as the primary control of the blood sugar. Either way, it's probably still a great idea to get your day started off right and add a few tablespoons to some juice in the morning.

8 BEST TYPES OF CARDIO FOR WEIGHT LOSS IN NO PARTICULAR ORDER

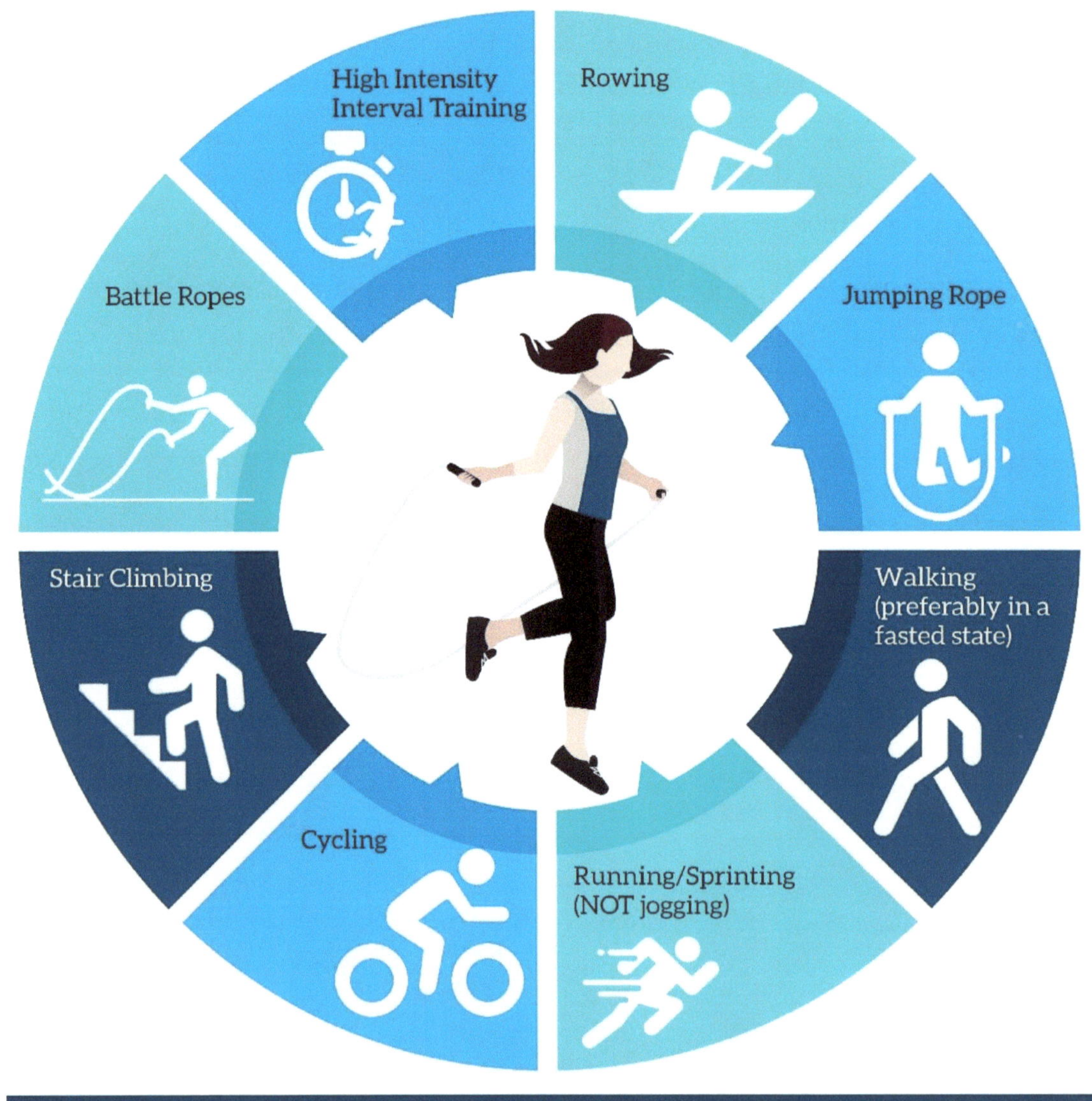

12-Week New Year Weight Loss Journal

https://www.amazon.com/gp/product/179046952X

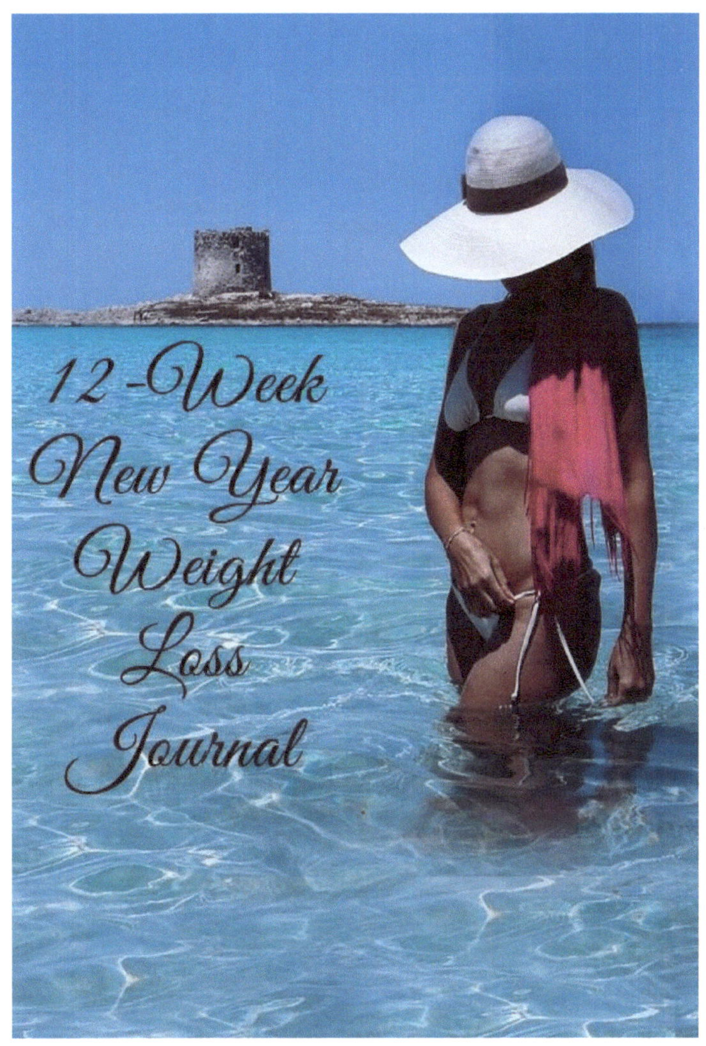

Now that the Holidays are over, one of your goals for the New Year may be to take off those pounds you gained over the holiday period - Thanksgiving through New Year's Day. That is the purpose of this weight loss journal and why it is for 12-weeks.

However if you stay the course over the 12-weeks, you will also have instilled your eating and workout routines as habits and can continue if you want. Just purchase another 12-week journal and continue where you left off.

As you go through the journal, you will first find a page to record your starting measurements, weight loss start date, and your personal goals for this journey. Be specific- don't say something like "I want to lose weight". It must be measurable, realistic and attainable. Something like "I want to lose 5 pounds a month". Or "I want to lose 1 1/2 to 2 pounds per week". With a 2-pound per week goal, you should lose around 24 pounds over the 12-week journey. Next you will find a series of worksheets – a set for each of the 12 weeks:

- A Shopping List

- A Meal Planner

– Two pages to cover the 7 days in each week

- 7 Daily Workout Sheets- A Progress Tracker

- A Lined Page to journal your thoughts, feelings, emotions, successes, failures, setbacks or anything you want to get down on paper.

Journaling can be a great way to identify trends you see that either work for you and should be continued, or ones that are holding you back and should be discarded. At the end of each month is a Progress Tracker to record your measurements again to see how they changed over that month. At the end of the journal is a page to record your total loss over the course of the 12-week journey.

Using a journal in conjunction with the book is a great way to stay accountable to your weight loss program and to record your progress.

New Me Weight Loss Journal

https://www.amazon.com/gp/product/1790687683

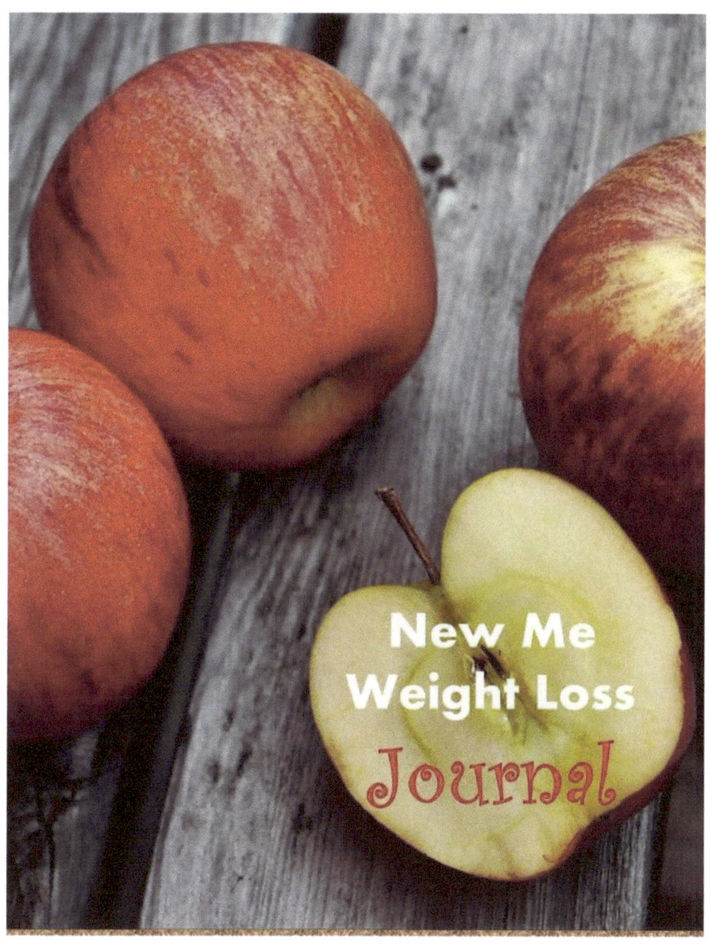

This 12-week journal starts off with a two-page explanation about the journal. Then a page to post a "before" photo and a page to record your Starting Body Measurements.

Next comes the set of pages for each week. The set begins with a two-page week with space to write in notes. After that comes a page with space to journal thoughts, feelings emotions and anything else you would like to get down on paper. That page also has a prompt at the bottom to spur writing thoughts.

Next comes a To Do List followed by Meal Plan and Food Diary pages to record the nutrition side of your weight loss plan followed by a Weight Tracker page. Now we move onto the exercise side with a Workout Tracker page and Water Tracker page.

Finally, the week wraps up with a Notes page to journal your final thoughts about the week. Midway through the 12-weeks are another set of Photos and Body Measurements page to record your progress so far.

Also, at the end of the 12-weeks are a final set of Photo and Body Measurements. By comparing the starting and ending photos and measurements, you can see just how far you have come in your weight loss journey.

Either 12-week journal will work just fine as far as a companion journal to the book.

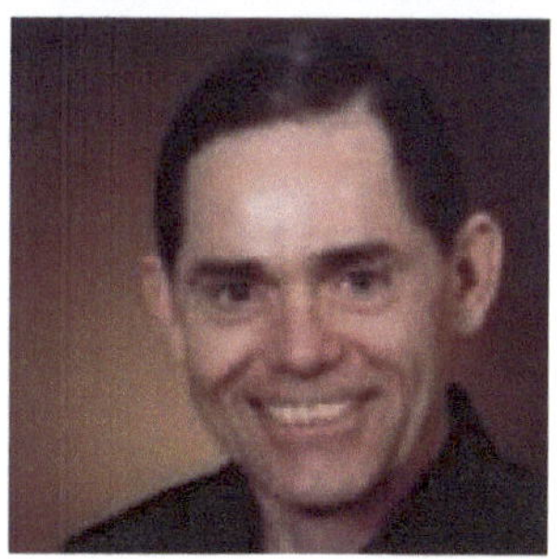

I have published numerous books on Amazon (both for Kindle and in paperback), along with other publishing platforms.

While most of my books are on health and fitness in general, I also write on baby boomer and older citizen health issues and have a recent interest in creating and printing journals/ planners and other printable products. A complete list of our published products on Amazon can be found at https://www.amazon.com/Ron-Kness/e/B0072M6PYO.

Besides my own writing, I also ghostwrite ebooks, books, reports, articles, blogs and do Kindle conversions for clients on a variety of topics. Contact me at Ron Kness Writing for a quote.

Today my wife and I are retired from our careers and live in Gold Canyon, AZ. I now write as a retirement business where you'll find me happily sitting in my office typing away on my laptop as I work on my next book or ghostwriting project . . . that is if we are not traveling on a cruise ship - our new-found mode of travel.